DEALING

A Journal of God's Promises

By Terri J. Fornear

DEALING WITH FEELINGS
A JOURNAL OF GOD'S PROMISES

© 2013 by Terri J. Fornear
ISBN: 978-0-9840113-2-2

Cover and book design by Rebecca Horn, rhorngraphics, rlrchorn@verizon.net

All rights reserved. No portion of this book may be reproduced or transmitted in any form or by any means, electronic or mechanical, without written permission of the author.

New American Standard Bible
Scripture quotations marked (NASB) are taken from the New American Standard Bible®, Copyright © 1960, 1962, 1963, 1968, 1971, 1972, 1973, 1975, 1977, 1995 by The Lockman Foundation. Used by permission. (www.Lockman.org)

New International Version
Scripture quotations marked (NIV) are taken from The Holy Bible, New International Version®, NIV®. Copyright © 1973, 1978, 1984 by Biblica, Inc.™ All rights reserved worldwide. (www.zondervan.com)

Amplified Bible
Scripture quotations marked (AMP) are taken from the Amplified® Bible, Copyright © 1954, 1958, 1962, 1964, 1965, 1987 by The Lockman Foundation. Used by permission. (www.Lockman.org)

Contemporary English Version
Scripture quotations marked (CEV) are from the Contemporary English Version Copyright © 1991, 1992, 1995 by American Bible Society, Used by Permission.

Good News Translation
Scripture quotations marked (GNT) are from the Good News Translation in Today's English Version- Second Edition Copyright © 1992 by American Bible Society. Used by Permission.

THE MESSAGE
Scripture quotations marked (THE MESSAGE) are from *THE MESSAGE*. Copyright © by Eugene H. Peterson 1993, 1994, 1995, 1996, 2000, 2001, 2002. Used by permission of NavPress Publishing Group.

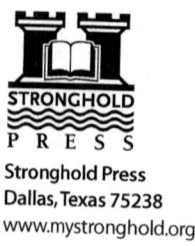

Stronghold Press
Dallas, Texas 75238
www.mystronghold.org

DEALING WITH FEELINGS

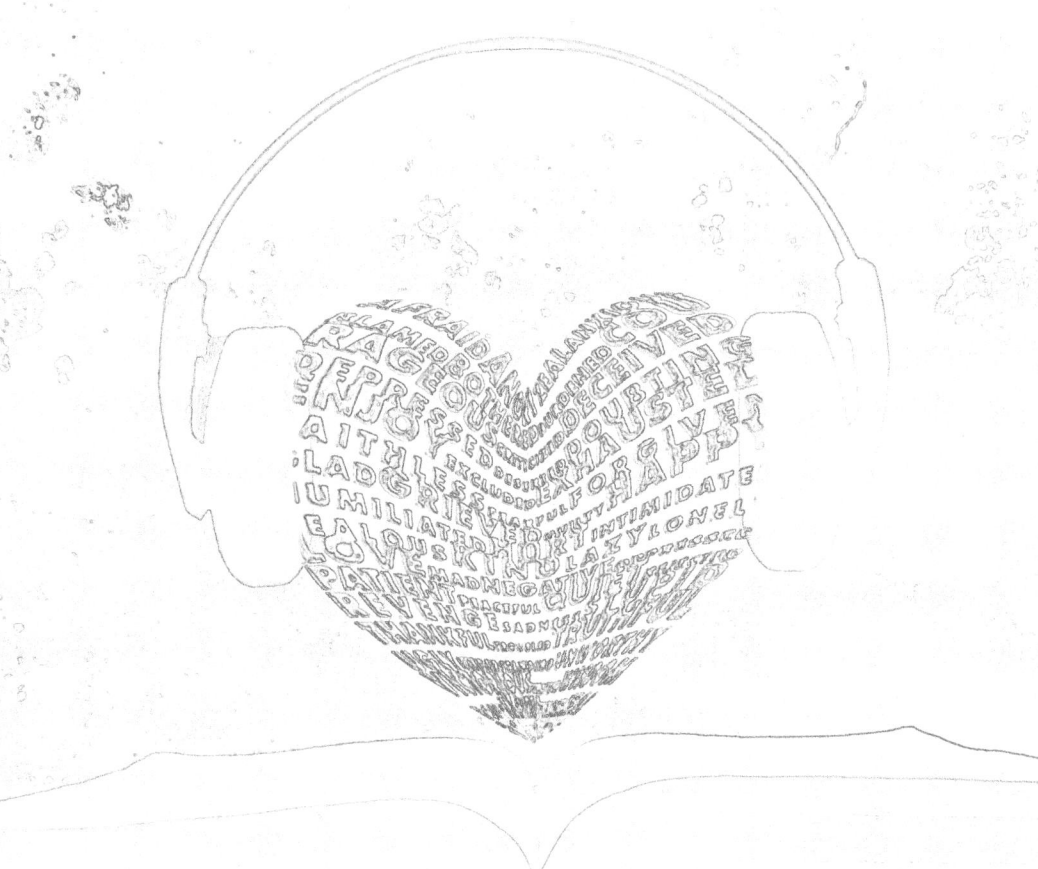

A JOURNAL
OF
GOD'S PROMISES

How To Use Dealing with Feelings

God has many promises for us. Our job is to ask and seek Him to receive them. He gave us a kind of emergency alarm in our body that goes off when we need a promise. This alarm is called our emotions. This book was written to help you recognize your emotions, and then receive God's great promises to meet your needs. You will find journal pages throughout this book which will help you to write down and deal with your feelings.

☑ **Step one** is to realize what causes the alarm to go off in your body. Describe what happened in the "Situation" space on the journal page. For example:

Situation: *The teacher pointed out in front of the whole class that I did not do my homework.*

☑ **Step two** is naming the **feeling or feelings** you have from the situation. For example:

Feelings: *You feel "stupid" that you forgot your homework because you hurried out of the house without it. You are upset because the teacher told the whole class.*

☑ **Step three** is knowing how that feeling makes you think about yourself. This is where a lie can creep in. Write down a conclusion you are tempted to make about yourself. For example:

Lie that creeps in: *Everybody thinks I am stupid. No one will want to be my friend. The teacher does not like me.*

☑ **Step four** is the most important. You need to know how and what God thinks of you. Look up the feelings under "stupid." The promise is:

What does God really think of you? Romans 8:38-39: *For I am convinced that neither death, nor life, nor angels, nor principalities, nor things present, nor things to come, nor powers, nor height, nor depth, nor any other created thing, will be able to separate us from the love of God, which is in Christ Jesus our Lord. (NASB)*

Keep reminding yourself of God's promise and stop listening to the lies. Writing down your feelings and believing God's view of you will change your feelings over time. Of course, you need to get your homework to your teacher on time. When you do make a mistake, you should not look at yourself through eyes of condemnation and fear, but through the eyes of the One who created you. He knows your weaknesses and still really loves you. The Bible calls this "renewing your mind" with God's thoughts about you.

—Terri Fornear

Romans 12:1-2
So here's what I want you to do, God helping you: Take your everyday, ordinary life—your sleeping, eating, going-to-work, and walking-around life—and place it before God as an offering. Embracing what God does for you is the best thing you can do for Him. Don't become so well-adjusted to your culture that you fit into it without even thinking. Instead, fix your attention on God. You'll be changed from the inside out. Readily recognize what He wants from you, and quickly respond to it. Unlike the culture around you, always dragging you down to its level of immaturity, God brings the best out, develops well-formed maturity in you. (THE MESSAGE)

Table of Contents

Afraid	6	Lazy	60
Angry	8	Lonely	62
Anxious	10	Love	64
Blamed	12	Mad	66
Bothered	14	Negative	68
Burdened	16	Oppressed	70
Courageous	18	Patient	72
Criticized	20	Peaceful	74
Deceived	22	Pressured	76
Depressed	24	Quiet	78
Deserted	26	Rejected	80
Doubting	28	Revenge	82
Enjoy	30	Sadness	84
Excluded	32	Stupid	86
Exhausted	34	Thankful	88
Faithless	36	Troubled	90
Fearful	38	Truthful	92
Forgiven	40	Ugly	94
Glad	42	Understanding	96
Grieved	44	Unworthy	98
Guilty	46	Victorious	100
Happy	48	Waiting	102
Humiliated	50	Wisdom	104
Hurt	52	Worry	106
Intimidated	54	eXcited	108
Jealous	56	Yielded	110
Kind	58	Zeal	112

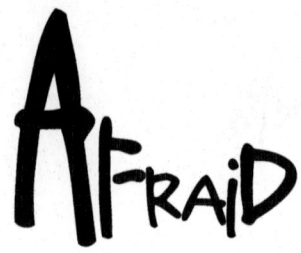

Afraid

Deuteronomy 31:6
Be strong and courageous, do not be afraid or tremble at them, for the LORD your God is the one who goes with you. He will not fail you or forsake you. (NASB)

Psalm 3:6
Ten thousand enemies attack from every side, but I am not afraid. (CEV)

Psalm 56:3
When I am afraid, O Lord Almighty, I put my trust in You. (GNT)

Psalm 91:5
You need not fear any dangers at night or sudden attacks during the day. (GNT)

Psalm 56:4
In God, whose word I praise, in God I have put my trust; I shall not be afraid. What can mere man do to me? (NASB)

Situation:

Feelings:

The lies that creep in about God:

What GOD thinks of you:

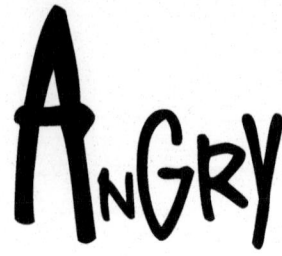

Angry

Proverbs 29:22
An angry person stirs up conflict, and a hot-tempered person commits many sins. (NIV)

Ecclesiastes 5:6
Don't let your mouth get you in trouble! (CEV)

Ecclesiastes 7:9
Keep your temper under control; it is foolish to harbor a grudge. (GNT)

Ephesians 4:26
When angry, do not sin; do not ever let your wrath (your exasperation, your fury or indignation) last until the sun goes down. (AMP)

James 1:19-20
My dear brothers and sisters, take note of this: Everyone should be quick to listen, slow to speak and slow to become angry, because human anger does not produce the righteousness that God desires. (NIV)

Situation:

Feelings:

The lies that creep in about God:

What GOD thinks of you:

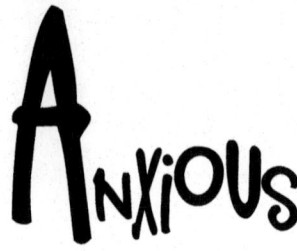

Anxious

Psalm 94:19
Whenever I am anxious and worried, You comfort me and make me glad. (GNT)

Philippians 4:6
Don't worry about anything, but pray about everything. With thankful hearts offer up your prayers and requests to God. (CEV)

Isaiah 35:4
Tell fearful souls, "Courage! Take heart! GOD is here, right here, on His way to put things right and redress all wrongs. He's on His way! He'll save you! (THE MESSAGE)

Proverbs 12:25
Worry is a heavy burden, but a kind word always brings cheer. (CEV)

1 Peter 5:7
Casting the whole of your care [all your anxieties, all your worries, all your concerns, once and for all] on Him, for He cares for you affectionately and cares about you watchfully. (AMP)

Situation:

_____
_____
_____
_____
_____

Feelings:

_____
_____
_____
_____
_____
_____

The lies that creep in about God:

_____
_____
_____
_____
_____
_____

What GOD thinks of you:

_____
_____
_____
_____
_____
_____
_____
_____

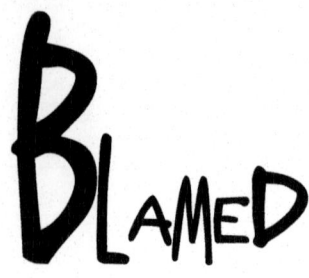

Romans 8:1
Therefore there is now no condemnation for those who are in Christ Jesus. (NASB)

Romans 4:7-8
Happy are those whose wrongs are forgiven, whose sins are pardoned! Happy is the person whose sins the Lord will not keep account of! (GNT)

Exodus 23:22
But if you obey Him and do everything I command, I will fight against all your enemies. (GNT)

Luke 6:27-28
But I say to you who hear, love your enemies, do good to those who hate you, bless those who curse you, pray for those who mistreat you. (NASB)

Psalm 13:2
How long must I be confused and miserable all day? How long will my enemies keep beating me down? (CEV)

Situation:

Feelings:

The lies that creep in about God:

What GOD thinks of you:

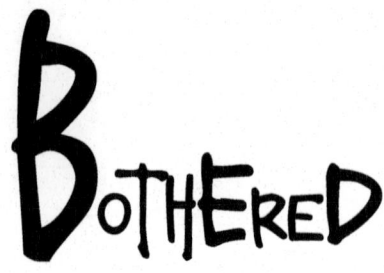

Bothered

John 14:27
Peace is what I leave with you; it is My own peace that I give you. I do not give it as the world does. Do not be worried and upset; do not be afraid. (GNT)

Matthew 6:25
Therefore I tell you, do not worry about your life, what you will eat or drink; or about your body, what you will wear. Is not life more than food, and the body more than clothes? (NIV)

Matthew 6:28
Why worry about clothes? Look how the wild flowers grow. They don't work hard to make their clothes. (CEV)

John 14:18
I will not leave you like orphans; I will come back to you. (CEV)

Luke 10:41
But the Lord answered and said to her, "Martha, Martha, you are worried and bothered about so many things. (NASB)

Situation:

Feelings:

The lies that creep in about God:

What GOD thinks of you:

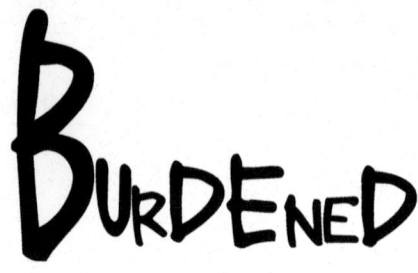

Burdened

Mathew 11:28
Come to me, all you who are weary and burdened, and I will give you rest. Take My yoke upon you and learn from Me, for I am gentle and humble in heart, and you will find rest for your souls. For My yoke is easy and My burden is light. (NIV)

Psalm 37:7
Be patient and wait for the Lord to act; don't be worried about those who prosper or those who succeed in their evil plans. (GNT)

Hebrews 4:9-10
As it is, however, there still remains for God's people a rest like God's resting on the seventh day. For those who receive that rest which God promised will rest from their own work, just as God rested from His. (GNT)

Psalms 46:10
Cease striving and know that I am God; I will be exalted among the nations, I will be exalted in the earth. (NASB)

1 Chronicles 29:11
Yours, O LORD, is the greatness and the power and the glory and the victory and the majesty, indeed everything that is in the heavens and the earth; Yours is the dominion, O LORD, and You exalt Yourself as head over all. (NASB)

Situation:

Feelings:

The lies that creep in about God:

What GOD thinks of you:

Courageous

John 16:33
These things I have spoken to you, so that in Me you may have peace. In the world you have tribulation, but take courage; I have overcome the world. (NASB)

Deuteronomy 31:6
Be strong and courageous. Do not be afraid or terrified because of them, for the Lord your God goes with you; He will never leave you nor forsake you. (NIV)

Joshua 10:25
Then Joshua said to his officers, "Don't be afraid or discouraged. Be determined and confident because this is what the Lord is going to do to all your enemies." (GNT)

1 Chronicles 28:20
Also David told Solomon his son, "Be strong and courageous, and do it. Fear not, be not dismayed, for the Lord God, my God, is with you. He will not fail or forsake you until you have finished all the work for the service of the house of the Lord." (AMP)

2 Chronicles 32:7
Be strong and courageous. Do not be afraid or discouraged because of the king of Assyria and the vast army with him, for there is a greater power with us than with him. (NIV)

Situation:

_____
_____
_____
_____
_____

Feelings:

_____
_____
_____
_____
_____

The lies that creep in about God:

_____
_____
_____
_____
_____

What GOD thinks of you:

_____
_____
_____
_____
_____
_____
_____

Criticized

Isaiah 54:17
"No weapon that is formed against you will prosper; and every tongue that accuses you in judgment you will condemn. This is the heritage of the servants of the LORD, and their vindication is from Me," declares the LORD. (NASB)

1 Corinthians 4:13
When they spread rumors about us, we put in a good word for them. (THE MESSAGE)

1 Peter 3:9
Do not pay back evil with evil or cursing with cursing; instead, pay back with a blessing, because a blessing is what God promised to give you when He called you. (GNT)

Proverbs 17:20
He who has a crooked mind finds no good, and he who is perverted in his language falls into evil. (NASB)

James 3:9-10
With the tongue we praise our Lord and Father, and with it we curse men, who have been made in God's likeness. Out of the same mouth come praise and cursing. My brothers, this should not be. (NIV)

Situation:

Feelings:

The lies that creep in about God:

What GOD thinks of you:

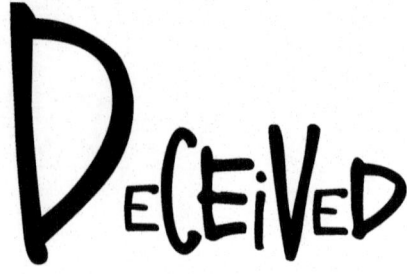

Deceived

1 Corinthians 15:33
Do not be so deceived and misled! Evil companionships (communion, associations) corrupt and deprave good manners and morals and character. (AMP)

2 Corinthians 11:3
But I am afraid that just as Eve was deceived by the serpent's cunning, your minds may somehow be led astray from your sincere and pure devotion to Christ. (NIV)

Galatians 6:7
Do not be deceived, God is not mocked; for whatever a man sows, this he will also reap. (NASB)

James 1:16-17
Do not be deceived, my dear friends! Every good gift and every perfect present comes from heaven; it comes down from God, the Creator of the heavenly lights, Who does not change or cause darkness by turning. (GNT)

Proverbs 24:28
Don't give evidence against others without good reason, or say misleading things about them. (GNT)

Situation:

Feelings:

The lies that creep in about God:

What GOD thinks of you:

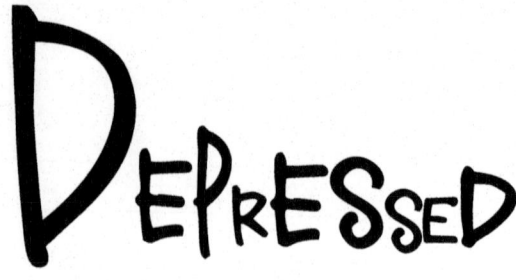

Depressed

2 Corinthians 7:6
But God, Who comforts and encourages and refreshes and cheers the depressed and the sinking, comforted and encouraged and refreshed and cheered us by the arrival of Titus. (AMP)

2 Corinthians 1:3-4
Blessed be the God and Father of our Lord Jesus Christ, the Father of mercies and God of all comfort, Who comforts us in all our affliction so that we will be able to comfort those who are in any affliction with the comfort with which we ourselves are comforted by God. (NASB)

Isaiah 61:1-3
The Spirit of the Sovereign LORD is on Me, because the LORD has anointed Me to preach good news to the poor. He has sent Me to bind up the brokenhearted, to proclaim freedom for the captives and release from darkness for the prisoners, to proclaim the year of the LORD's favor and the day of vengeance of our God, to comfort all who mourn, and provide for those who grieve in Zion—to bestow on them a crown of beauty instead of ashes, the oil of gladness instead of mourning, and a garment of praise instead of a spirit of despair. They will be called oaks of righteousness, a planting of the LORD for the display of His splendor. (NASB)

Psalms 51:17
I learned God-worship when my pride was shattered. Heart-shattered lives ready for love don't for a moment escape God's notice. (THE MESSAGE)

Hebrews 13:5-6
Keep your lives free from the love of money, and be satisfied with what you have. For God has said, "I will never leave you; I will never abandon you." (GNT)

Situation:

_____
_____
_____
_____
_____

Feelings:

_____
_____
_____
_____
_____

The lies that creep in about God:

_____
_____
_____
_____
_____

What GOD thinks of you:

_____
_____
_____
_____
_____
_____
_____

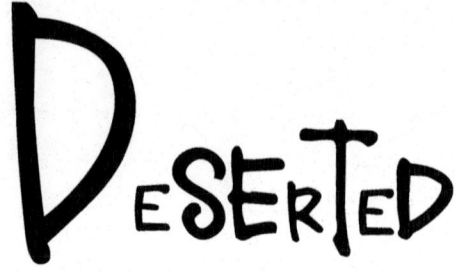

Psalm 25:16
Turn to me, Lord, and be merciful to me, because I am lonely and weak. (GNT)

Psalm 68:6
God makes a home for the lonely; He leads out the prisoners into prosperity. Only the rebellious dwell in a parched land. (NASB)

1 Samuel 12:22
God, simply because of who He is, is not going to walk off and leave His people. God took delight in making you into His very own people. (THE MESSAGE)

Psalm 42:5
Why are you in despair, O my soul? And why have you become disturbed within me? Hope in God, for I shall again praise Him for the help of His presence. (NASB)

Psalms 37:25
I am old now; I have lived a long time, but I have never seen good people abandoned by the Lord or their children begging for food. (GNT)

Situation:

Feelings:

The lies that creep in about God:

What GOD thinks of you:

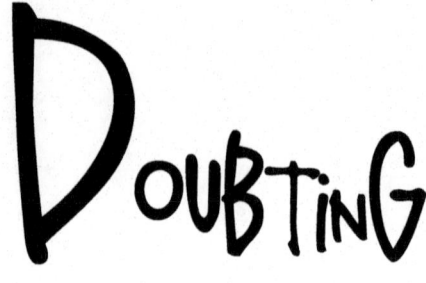

Doubting

James 1:5-6
But if any of you lack wisdom, you should pray to God, Who will give it to you; because God gives generously and graciously to all. But when you pray, you must believe and not doubt at all. Whoever doubts is like a wave in the sea that is driven and blown about by the wind. (GNT)

Jude 1:22
Be helpful to all who may have doubts. (CEV)

Mark 11:22-24
And Jesus answered saying to them, "Have faith in God. Truly I say to you, whoever says to this mountain, 'Be taken up and cast into the sea,' and does not doubt in his heart, but believes that what he says is going to happen, it will be granted him. Therefore I say to you, all things for which you pray and ask, believe that you have received them, and they will be granted you. (NASB)

Matthew 14:28-32
Then Peter spoke up. "Lord, if it is really You, order me to come out on the water to You." "Come!" answered Jesus. So Peter got out of the boat and started walking on the water to Jesus. But when he noticed the strong wind, he was afraid and started to sink down in the water. "Save me, Lord!" he cried. At once Jesus reached out and grabbed hold of him and said, "What little faith you have! Why did you doubt?" They both got into the boat, and the wind died down. (GNT)

Hebrews 12:2-3
Keep your eyes on Jesus, Who both began and finished this race we're in. Study how He did it. Because He never lost sight of where He was headed—that exhilarating finish in and with God—He could put up with anything along the way: cross, shame, whatever. And now He's there, in the place of honor, right alongside God. When you find yourselves flagging in your faith, go over that story again, item by item, that long litany of hostility He plowed through. (THE MESSAGE)

Situation:

Feelings:

The lies that creep in about God:

What GOD thinks of you:

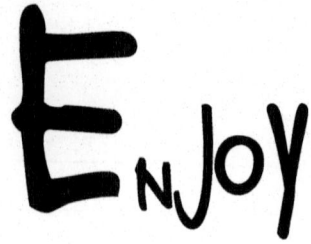

Psalm 16:11
You will make known to me the path of life; in Your presence is fullness of joy; in Your right hand there are pleasures forever. (NASB)

Psalm 5:11
But let all who take refuge in You be glad; let them ever sing for joy. Spread Your protection over them, that those who love Your name may rejoice in You. (NIV)

Psalm 20:5
Then you will win victories, and we will celebrate, while raising our banners in the name of our God. May the Lord answer all of your prayers! (CEV)

Psalm 92:4
For You, O LORD, have made me glad by what You have done, I will sing for joy at the works of Your hands. (NASB)

Psalm 95:1-3
O come, let us sing for joy to the Lord, let us shout joyfully to the rock of our salvation. Let us come before His presence with thanksgiving, let us shout joyfully to Him with psalms. For the Lord is a great God and a great King above all gods. (NASB)

Situation:

Feelings:

The lies that creep in about God:

What GOD thinks of you:

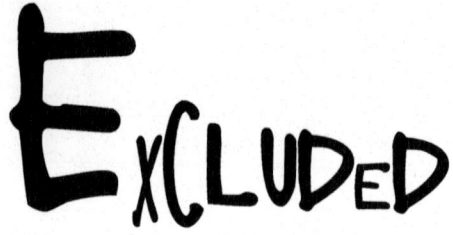

1 Peter 2:4
Come to Jesus Christ. He is the living stone that people have rejected, but which God has chosen and highly honored. (CEV)

John 15:9
I've loved you the way My Father has loved Me. Make yourselves at home in My love. (THE MESSAGE)

Romans 8:28
And we know that God causes all things to work together for good to those who love God, to those who are called according to His purpose. (NASB)

John 12:42-43
Even then, many Jewish authorities believed in Jesus; but because of the Pharisees they did not talk about it openly, so as not to be expelled from the synagogue. They loved human approval rather than the approval of God. (GNT)

Colossians 3:12
God loves you and has chosen you as His own special people. So be gentle, kind, humble, meek, and patient. (CEV)

Situation:

_____
_____
_____
_____
_____

Feelings:

_____
_____
_____
_____
_____
_____

The lies that creep in about God:

_____
_____
_____
_____
_____
_____

What GOD thinks of you:

_____
_____
_____
_____
_____
_____
_____
_____

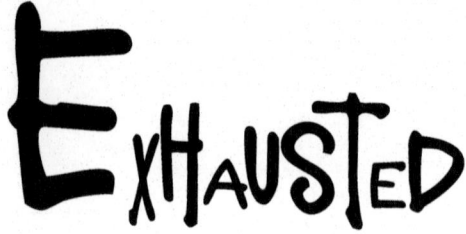

Isaiah 40:28-31
Don't you know? Haven't you heard? The Lord is the eternal God, Creator of the earth. He never gets weary or tired; His wisdom cannot be measured. The Lord gives strength to those who are weary. Even young people get tired, then stumble and fall. But those who trust the Lord will find new strength. They will be strong like eagles soaring upward on wings; they will walk and run without getting tired. (CEV)

2 Corinthians 12:8-10
Three times I pleaded with the Lord to take it away from me. But He said to me, "My grace is sufficient for you, for My power is made perfect in weakness." Therefore I will boast all the more gladly about my weaknesses, so that Christ's power may rest on me. That is why, for Christ's sake, I delight in weaknesses, in insults, in hardships, in persecutions, in difficulties. For when I am weak, then I am strong. (NIV)

Ephesians 1:18-21
I pray that the eyes of your heart may be enlightened, so that you will know what is the hope of His calling, what are the riches of the glory of His inheritance in the saints, and what is the surpassing greatness of His power toward us who believe. These are in accordance with the working of the strength of His might which He brought about in Christ, when He raised Him from the dead and seated Him at His right hand in the heavenly places, far above all rule and authority and power and dominion, and every name that is named, not only in this age but also in the one to come. (NASB)

Ephesians 3:16-17
I ask Him to strengthen you by His Spirit—not a brute strength but a glorious inner strength—that Christ will live in you as you open the door and invite Him in. (THE MESSAGE)

2 Corinthians 4:7
But we have this treasure in earthen vessels, so that the surpassing greatness of the power will be of God and not from ourselves. (NASB)

Situation:

Feelings:

The lies that creep in about God:

What GOD thinks of you:

Faithless

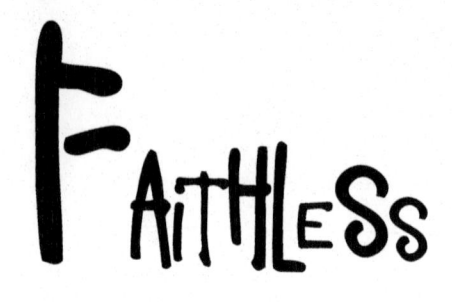

Hosea 6:1-3
Come, let us return to the LORD. For He has torn us, but He will heal us; He has wounded us, but He will bandage us. He will revive us after two days; He will raise us up on the third day, that we may live before Him. So let us know, let us press on to know the LORD. His going forth is as certain as the dawn; and He will come to us like the rain, like the spring rain watering the earth. (NASB)

Proverbs 28:13
Whoever conceals their sins does not prosper, but the one who confesses and renounces them finds mercy. (NIV)

1 John 1:9
If we [freely] admit that we have sinned and confess our sins, He is faithful and just (true to His own nature and promises) and will forgive our sins [dismiss our lawlessness] and [continuously] cleanse us from all unrighteousness [everything not in conformity to His will in purpose, thought, and action]. (AMP)

Philippians 3:12-14
Not that I have already obtained it or have already become perfect, but I press on so that I may lay hold of that for which also I was laid hold of by Christ Jesus. Brethren, I do not regard myself as having laid hold of it yet; but one thing I do: forgetting what lies behind and reaching forward to what lies ahead, I press on toward the goal for the prize of the upward call of God in Christ Jesus. (NASB)

2 Timothy 2:13
If we are not faithful, He remains faithful, because He cannot be false to Himself. (GNT)

Situation:

Feelings:

The lies that creep in about God:

What GOD thinks of you:

Fearful

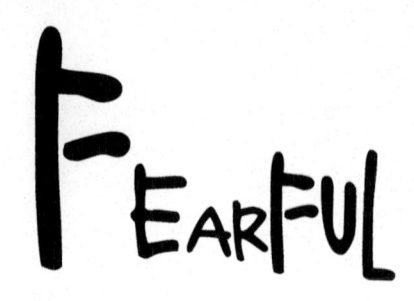

Psalm 23:4
Even though I walk through the valley of the shadow of death, I fear no evil, for You are with me; Your rod and Your staff, they comfort me. (NASB)

John 14:27
Peace I leave with you; My [own] peace I now give and bequeath to you. Not as the world gives do I give to you. Do not let your hearts be troubled, neither let them be afraid. [Stop allowing yourselves to be agitated and disturbed; and do not permit yourselves to be fearful and intimidated and cowardly and unsettled.] (AMP)

Psalm 27:1
The Lord is my light and my salvation—whom shall I fear? The Lord is the stronghold of my life—of whom shall I be afraid? (NIV)

1 John 4:18
There is no room in love for fear. Well-formed love banishes fear. Since fear is crippling, a fearful life—fear of death, fear of judgment—is one not yet fully formed in love. (THE MESSAGE)

2 Timothy 1:7
For the Spirit that God has given us does not make us timid; instead, His Spirit fills us with power, love, and self-control. (GNT)

Situation:

Feelings:

The lies that creep in about God:

What GOD thinks of you:

Forgiven

1 John 2:1-2
My dear children, I write this to you so that you will not sin. But if anybody does sin, we have One who speaks to the Father in our defense—Jesus Christ, the Righteous One. He is the atoning sacrifice for our sins, and not only for ours but also for the sins of the whole world. (NIV)

Romans 4:5-8
But you cannot make God accept you because of something you do. God accepts sinners only because they have faith in Him. In the Scriptures, David talks about the blessings that come to people who are acceptable to God, even though they don't do anything to deserve these blessings. David says, "God blesses people whose sins are forgiven and whose evil deeds are forgotten. The Lord blesses people whose sins are erased from His book." (CEV)

Ephesians 4:32
Be kind to one another, tender-hearted, forgiving each other, just as God in Christ also has forgiven you. (NASB)

2 Chronicles 7:14
If My people, who are called by My name, will humble themselves and pray and seek My face and turn from their wicked ways, then will I hear from heaven and will forgive their sin and will heal their land. (NASB)

Luke 17:4
If he sins against you seven times in one day, and each time he comes to you saying, "I repent," you must forgive him. (GNT)

Situation:

Feelings:

The lies that creep in about God:

What GOD thinks of you:

Glad

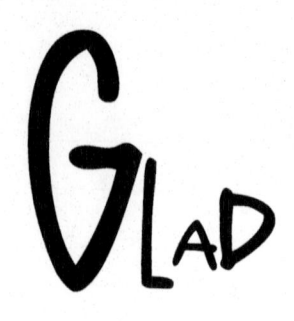

Psalm 31:7
I will be glad and rejoice in Your mercy and steadfast love, because You have seen my affliction, You have taken note of my life's distresses. (AMP)

Psalms 90:15
Make us glad according to the days You have afflicted us, and the years we have seen evil. (NASB)

James 1:2-4
My friends, be glad, even if you have a lot of trouble. You know that you learn to endure by having your faith tested. But you must learn to endure everything, so that you will be completely mature and not lacking in anything. (CEV)

Psalm 40:16
Our Lord, let Your worshipers rejoice and be glad. They love You for saving them, so let them always say, "The Lord is wonderful!" (CEV)

Revelation 19:6-7
Then I heard what sounded like a great multitude, like the roar of rushing waters and like loud peals of thunder, shouting: "Hallelujah! For our Lord God Almighty reigns. Let us rejoice and be glad and give Him glory! For the wedding of the Lamb has come, and His bride has made herself ready." (NIV)

Situation:

_____
_____
_____
_____
_____

Feelings:

_____
_____
_____
_____
_____

The lies that creep in about God:

_____
_____
_____
_____
_____

What GOD thinks of you:

_____
_____
_____
_____
_____
_____

GRIEVED

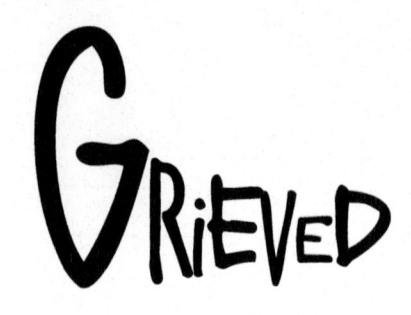

John 16:20
Very truly I tell you, you will weep and mourn while the world rejoices. You will grieve, but your grief will turn to joy. (NIV)

Job 1:20-22
Then Job got up and tore his clothes in grief. He shaved his head and threw himself face downward on the ground. He said, "I was born with nothing, and I will die with nothing. The Lord gave, and now He has taken away. May His name be praised!" In spite of everything that had happened, Job did not sin by blaming God. (GNT)

Habakkuk 3:17-18
Even though the fig trees have no fruit and no grapes grow on the vines, even though the olive crop fails and the fields produce no grain, even though the sheep all die and the cattle stalls are empty, I will still be joyful and glad, because the Lord God is my savior. (GNT)

Psalm 119:28
My soul weeps because of grief. Strengthen me according to Your word. (NASB)

Psalm 30:5
For His anger is but for a moment, His favor is for a lifetime; weeping may last for the night, but a shout of joy comes in the morning. (NASB)

Situation:

Feelings:

The lies that creep in about God:

What GOD thinks of you:

Guilty

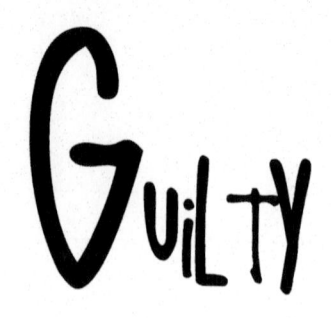

Romans 8:1
Therefore, there is now no condemnation for those who are in Christ Jesus. (NIV)

Hebrews 10:11-13
Every Jewish priest performs his services every day and offers the same sacrifices many times; but these sacrifices can never take away sins. Christ, however, offered one sacrifice for sins, an offering that is effective forever, and then He sat down at the right side of God. There He now waits until God puts His enemies as a footstool under His feet. (GNT)

2 Corinthians 5:17
Anyone who belongs to Christ is a new person. The past is forgotten, and everything is new. (CEV)

Revelation 12:10-11
Then I heard a strong voice out of Heaven saying, "Salvation and power are established! Kingdom of our God, authority of His Messiah! The Accuser of our brothers and sisters thrown out, who accused them day and night before God. They defeated him through the blood of the Lamb and the bold word of their witness. They weren't in love with themselves; they were willing to die for Christ." (THE MESSAGE)

Luke 7:47
For this reason I say to you, her sins, which are many, have been forgiven, for she loved much; but he who is forgiven little, loves little. (NASB)

Situation:

Feelings:

The lies that creep in about God:

What GOD thinks of you:

Happy

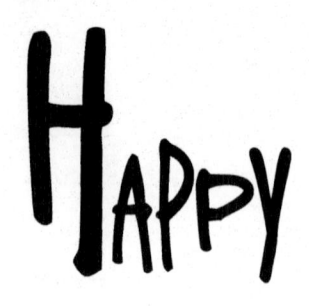

Psalm 1:1-3
Happy are those who reject the advice of evil people, who do not follow the example of sinners or join those who have no use for God. Instead, they find joy in obeying the Law of the Lord, and they study it day and night. They are like trees that grow beside a stream, that bear fruit at the right time, and whose leaves do not dry up. They succeed in everything they do. (GNT)

1 Thessalonians 5:16-18
Be cheerful no matter what; pray all the time; thank God no matter what happens. This is the way God wants you who belong to Christ Jesus to live. (THE MESSAGE)

Ecclesiastes 7:14
When things are going well for you, be glad, and when trouble comes, just remember: God sends both happiness and trouble; you never know what is going to happen next. (GNT)

Ecclesiastes 5:19
Moreover, when God gives someone wealth and possessions, and the ability to enjoy them, to accept their lot and be happy in their toil—this is a gift of God. (NIV)

Hebrews 12:9-11
Moreover, we have all had human fathers who disciplined us and we respected them for it. How much more should we submit to the Father of our spirits and live! Our fathers disciplined us for a little while as they thought best; but God disciplines us for our good, that we may share in His holiness. No discipline seems pleasant at the time, but painful. Later on, however, it produces a harvest of righteousness and peace for those who have been trained by it. (NIV)

Situation:

Feelings:

The lies that creep in about God:

What GOD thinks of you:

Humiliated

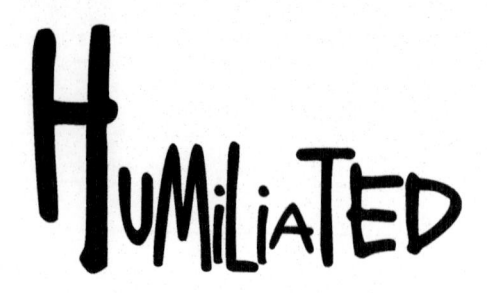

Psalms 27:1
The LORD is my light and my salvation; whom shall I fear? The LORD is the defense of my life; whom shall I dread? (NASB)

Romans 8:31-32
What then shall we say to these things? If God is for us, who is against us? He who did not spare His own Son, but delivered Him over for us all, how will He not also with Him freely give us all things? (NASB)

Colossians 2:9-10
For the full content of divine nature lives in Christ, in His humanity, and you have been given full life in union with Him. He is supreme over every spiritual ruler and authority. (GNT)

1 Peter 5:5-6
And you who are younger must follow your leaders. But all of you, leaders and followers alike, are to be down to earth with each other, for—God has had it with the proud, but takes delight in just plain people. So be content with who you are, and don't put on airs. God's strong hand is on you; He'll promote you at the right time. (THE MESSAGE)

Proverbs 3:34
He mocks proud mockers but shows favor to the humble and oppressed. (NIV)

Situation:

Feelings:

The lies that creep in about God:

What GOD thinks of you:

Hurt

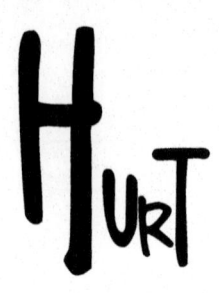

James 5:13
Is anyone among you afflicted (ill-treated, suffering evil)? He should pray. (AMP)

Matthew 5:11-12
Blessed are you when people insult you, persecute you and falsely say all kinds of evil against you because of Me. Rejoice and be glad, because great is your reward in heaven, for in the same way they persecuted the prophets who were before you. (NIV)

2 Corinthians 12:10
Therefore I am well content with weaknesses, with insults, with distresses, with persecutions, with difficulties, for Christ's sake; for when I am weak, then I am strong. (NASB)

1 Corinthians 13:4-5
Love is kind and patient, never jealous, boastful, proud, or rude. Love isn't selfish or quick tempered. It doesn't keep a record of wrongs that others do. (CEV)

1 Peter 3:8-9
Finally, all of you should agree and have concern and love for each other. You should also be kind and humble. Don't be hateful and insult people just because they are hateful and insult you. Instead, treat everyone with kindness. You are God's chosen ones, and He will bless you. (CEV)

Situation:

Feelings:

The lies that creep in about God:

What GOD thinks of you:

INTIMIDATED

Isaiah 51:7
Listen now, you who know right from wrong, you who hold My teaching inside you: Pay no attention to insults, and when mocked don't let it get you down. (THE MESSAGE)

1 Peter 3:14
Even if you have to suffer for doing good things, God will bless you. So stop being afraid and don't worry about what people might do. (CEV)

Acts 4:29-31
"And now they're at it again! Take care of their threats and give Your servants fearless confidence in preaching your Message, as You stretch out Your hand to us in healings and miracles and wonders done in the name of Your holy servant Jesus." While they were praying, the place where they were meeting trembled and shook. They were all filled with the Holy Spirit and continued to speak God's Word with fearless confidence. (THE MESSAGE)

Luke 12:4-5
I say to you, My friends, do not be afraid of those who kill the body and after that have no more that they can do. But I will warn you whom to fear: fear the One who, after He has killed, has authority to cast into hell; yes, I tell you, fear Him! (NASB)

Deuteronomy 31:8
The Lord Himself goes before you and will be with you; He will never leave you nor forsake you. Do not be afraid; do not be discouraged. (NIV)

Situation:

Feelings:

The lies that creep in about God:

What GOD thinks of you:

Jealous

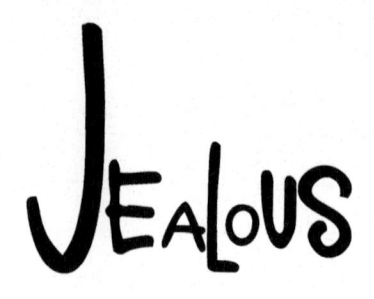

1 Corinthians 13:4
Love is patient, love is kind and is not jealous. (NASB)

Philippians 4:11-13
I am not saying this because I am in need, for I have learned to be content whatever the circumstances. I know what it is to be in need, and I know what it is to have plenty. I have learned the secret of being content in any and every situation, whether well fed or hungry, whether living in plenty or in want. I can do everything through Him Who gives me strength. (NIV)

Proverbs 24:1
Don't be envious of evil people, and don't try to make friends with them. (GNT)

James 4:1-3
Why do you fight and argue with each other? Isn't it because you are full of selfish desires that fight to control your body? You want something you don't have, and you will do anything to get it. You will even kill! But you still cannot get what you want, and you won't get it by fighting and arguing. You should pray for it. Yet even when you do pray, your prayers are not answered, because you pray just for selfish reasons. (CEV)

Psalm 23:1-6
The LORD is my shepherd, I shall not want. He makes me lie down in green pastures; He leads me beside quiet waters. He restores my soul; He guides me in the paths of righteousness for His name's sake. Even though I walk through the valley of the shadow of death, I fear no evil, for You are with me; Your rod and Your staff, they comfort me. You prepare a table before me in the presence of my enemies; You have anointed my head with oil; my cup overflows. Surely goodness and lovingkindness will follow me all the days of my life, and I will dwell in the house of the LORD forever. (NASB)

Situation:

Feelings:

The lies that creep in about God:

What GOD thinks of you:

Kind

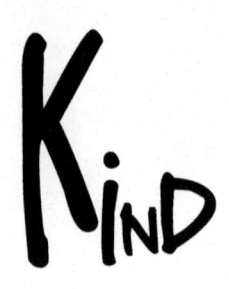

Micah 6:8
He has told you, O man, what is good; and what does the LORD require of you: But to do justice, to love kindness, and to walk humbly with your God? (NASB)

Proverbs 3:3-4
Do not let kindness and truth leave you; bind them around your neck, write them on the tablet of your heart. So you will find favor and good repute in the sight of God and man. (NASB)

Proverbs 25:21
If your enemy is hungry, give him bread to eat; and if he is thirsty, give him water to drink. (AMP)

Romans 12:21
Do not be overcome by evil, but overcome evil with good. (NIV)

Genesis 24:13-14
Behold, I am standing by the spring, and the daughters of the men of the city are coming out to draw water; now may it be that the girl to whom I say, "Please let down your jar so that I may drink," and who answers, "Drink, and I will water your camels also"—may she be the one whom You have appointed for Your servant Isaac; and by this I will know that You have shown lovingkindness to my master. (NASB)

Situation:

Feelings:

The lies that creep in about God:

What GOD thinks of you:

Lazy

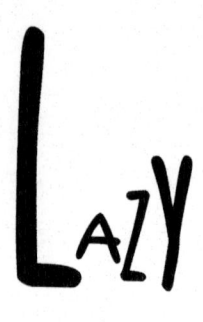

Proverbs 6:6-11
Go to the ant, O sluggard, observe her ways and be wise, which, having no chief, officer or ruler, prepares her food in the summer and gathers her provision in the harvest. How long will you lie down, O sluggard? When will you arise from your sleep? "A little sleep, a little slumber, a little folding of the hands to rest"—your poverty will come in like a vagabond and your need like an armed man. (NASB)

Proverbs 26:14-15
Lazy people turn over in bed. They get no farther than a door swinging on its hinges. Some people are too lazy to put food in their own mouths. (GNT)

2 Thessalonians 3:10-13
For even when we were with you, we gave you this rule: "The one who is unwilling to work shall not eat." We hear that some among you are idle and disruptive. They are not busy; they are busybodies. Such people we command and urge in the Lord Jesus Christ to settle down and earn the food they eat. And as for you, brothers and sisters, never tire of doing what is good. (NIV)

Proverbs 24:30-34
I once walked by the field and the vineyard of a lazy fool. Thorns and weeds were everywhere, and the stone wall had fallen down. When I saw this, it taught me a lesson: Sleep a little. Doze a little. Fold your hands and twiddle your thumbs. Suddenly poverty hits you and everything is gone! (CEV)

Proverbs 26:16
The sluggard is wiser in his own eyes than seven men who answer discreetly. (NIV)

Situation:

Feelings:

The lies that creep in about God:

What GOD thinks of you:

Lonely

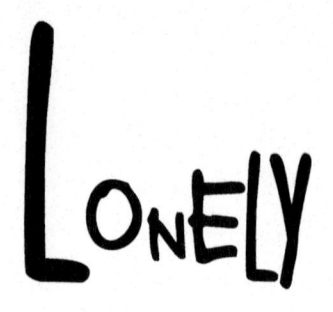

Psalm 22:1-5
My God, my God, why have You forsaken me? Why are You so far from saving me, so far from the words of my groaning? O my God, I cry out by day, but You do not answer, by night, but I find no rest. Yet You are enthroned as the Holy One; You are the praise of Israel. In You our fathers put their trust; they trusted and You delivered them. They cried to You and were saved; in You they trusted and were not disappointed. (NIV)

Isaiah 41:10
Don't panic. I'm with you. There's no need to fear for I'm your God. I'll give you strength. I'll help you. I'll hold you steady, keep a firm grip on you. (THE MESSAGE)

Psalm 68:4-6
Sing to God, sing praises to His name; lift up a song for Him Who rides through the deserts, Whose name is the LORD, and exult before Him. A father of the fatherless and a judge for the widows, is God in His holy habitation. God makes a home for the lonely; He leads out the prisoners into prosperity. (NASB)

Proverbs 18:24
One who has unreliable friends soon comes to ruin, but there is a friend who sticks closer than a brother. (NIV)

Psalm 16:11
You will show me the path of life; in Your presence is fullness of joy, at Your right hand there are pleasures forevermore. (AMP)

Situation:

Feelings:

The lies that creep in about God:

What GOD thinks of you:

LOVE

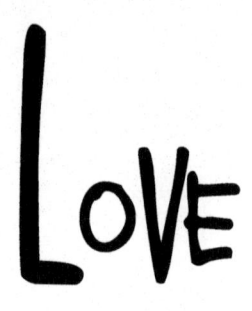

Romans 8:35-39
Who shall separate us from the love of Christ? Shall trouble or hardship or persecution or famine or nakedness or danger or sword? As it is written: "For Your sake we face death all day long; we are considered as sheep to be slaughtered." No, in all these things we are more than conquerors through Him who loved us. For I am convinced that neither death nor life, neither angels nor demons, neither the present nor the future, nor any powers, neither height nor depth, nor anything else in all creation, will be able to separate us from the love of God that is in Christ Jesus our Lord. (NIV)

Ephesians 3:16-19
That He would grant you, according to the riches of His glory, to be strengthened with power through His Spirit in the inner man, so that Christ may dwell in your hearts through faith; and that you, being rooted and grounded in love, may be able to comprehend with all the saints what is the breadth and length and height and depth, and to know the love of Christ which surpasses knowledge, that you may be filled up to all the fullness of God. (NASB)

1 John 4:19
We love because God first loved us. (GNT)

1 John 3:16-18
This is how we've come to understand and experience love: Christ sacrificed His life for us. This is why we ought to live sacrificially for our fellow believers, and not just be out for ourselves. If you see some brother or sister in need and have the means to do something about it but turn a cold shoulder and do nothing, what happens to God's love? It disappears. And you made it disappear. My dear children, let's not just talk about love; let's practice real love.

    Let us love, because God has sent His only begotten Son into the world, so that we might live through Him. (THE MESSAGE)

Situation:

Feelings:

The lies that creep in about God:

What GOD thinks of you:

MAD

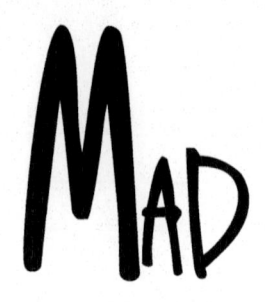

Proverbs 25:23
Gossip brings anger just as surely as the north wind brings rain. (GNT)

Proverbs 22:24-25
Do not make friends with a hot-tempered man, do not associate with one easily angered, or you may learn his ways and get yourself ensnared. (NIV)

Genesis 4:4-5
Abel, on his part also brought of the firstlings of his flock and of their fat portions. And the LORD had regard for Abel and for his offering; but for Cain and for his offering He had no regard. So Cain became very angry and his countenance fell. Then the LORD said to Cain, "Why are you angry? And why has your countenance fallen? If you do well, will not your countenance be lifted up? And if you do not do well, sin is crouching at the door; and its desire is for you, but you must master it." (NASB)

Psalm 37:8-11
Cease from anger and forsake wrath; do not fret; it leads only to evildoing. For evildoers will be cut off, but those who wait for the LORD, they will inherit the land. Yet a little while and the wicked man will be no more; and you will look carefully for his place and he will not be there. But the humble will inherit the land and will delight themselves in abundant prosperity. (NASB)

Ephesians 4:31
Stop being bitter and angry and mad at others. Don't yell at one another or curse each other or ever be rude. (CEV)

Situation:

Feelings:

The lies that creep in about God:

What GOD thinks of you:

Negative

Philippians 4:8
Finally, brethren, whatever is true, whatever is honorable, whatever is right, whatever is pure, whatever is lovely, whatever is of good repute, if there is any excellence and if anything worthy of praise, dwell on these things. (NASB)

Ephesians 5:7-10
Therefore do not be partners with them. For you were once darkness, but now you are light in the Lord. Live as children of light (for the fruit of the light consists in all goodness, righteousness and truth) and find out what pleases the Lord. (NIV)

Psalm 139:12
Even the darkness is not dark to You, and the night is as bright as the day. Darkness and light are alike to You. (NASB)

James 3:13-18
Who is wise and understanding among you? Let him show it by his good life, by deeds done in the humility that comes from wisdom. But if you harbor bitter envy and selfish ambition in your hearts, do not boast about it or deny the truth. Such "wisdom" does not come down from heaven but is earthly, unspiritual, of the devil. For where you have envy and selfish ambition, there you find disorder and every evil practice. But the wisdom that comes from heaven is first of all pure; then peace-loving, considerate, submissive, full of mercy and good fruit, impartial and sincere. Peacemakers who sow in peace raise a harvest of righteousness. (NIV)

Ephesians 5:4
Though some tongues just love the taste of gossip, Christians have better uses for language than that. Don't talk dirty or silly. That kind of talk doesn't fit our style. Thanksgiving is our dialect. (THE MESSAGE)

Situation:

Feelings:

The lies that creep in about God:

What GOD thinks of you:

Oppressed

Psalm 9:9
The LORD also will be a stronghold for the oppressed, a stronghold in times of trouble. (NASB)

Ephesians 6:11-13
Put on the full armor of God so that you can take your stand against the devil's schemes. For our struggle is not against flesh and blood, but against the rulers, against the authorities, against the powers of this dark world and against the spiritual forces of evil in the heavenly realms. Therefore put on the full armor of God, so that when the day of evil comes, you may be able to stand your ground, and after you have done everything, to stand. (NIV)

Psalm 103:6
The Lord executes righteousness and justice [not for me only, but] for all who are oppressed. (AMP)

Acts 10:38
You know of Jesus of Nazareth, how God anointed Him with the Holy Spirit and with power, and how He went about doing good and healing all who were oppressed by the devil, for God was with Him. (NASB)

Luke 4:18
The Spirit of the Lord is on Me, because He has anointed me to proclaim good news to the poor. He has sent me to proclaim freedom for the prisoners and recovery of sight for the blind, to set the oppressed free. (NIV)

Situation:

Feelings:

The lies that creep in about God:

What GOD thinks of you:

PATIENT

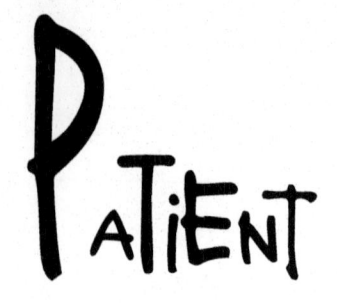

1 Corinthians 13:4
Love is patient; love is kind and is not jealous; love does not brag and is not arrogant. (NASB)

Galatians 5:22-23
But the Spirit produces love, joy, peace, patience, kindness, goodness, faithfulness, humility, and self-control. There is no law against such things as these. (GNT)

1 Thessalonians 5:14
And we earnestly beseech you, brethren, admonish (warn and seriously advise) those who are out of line [the loafers, the disorderly, and the unruly]; encourage the timid and fainthearted, help and give your support to the weak souls, [and] be very patient with everybody [always keeping your temper]. (AMP)

2 Timothy 2:24-26
The Lord's bond-servant must not be quarrelsome, but be kind to all, able to teach, patient when wronged, with gentleness correcting those who are in opposition, if perhaps God may grant them repentance leading to the knowledge of the truth, and they may come to their senses and escape from the snare of the devil, having been held captive by him to do his will. (NASB)

James 5:7-8
My friends, be patient until the Lord returns. Think of farmers who wait patiently for the spring and summer rains to make their valuable crops grow. Be patient like those farmers and don't give up. The Lord will soon be here! (CEV)

Situation:

Feelings:

The lies that creep in about God:

What GOD thinks of you:

Peaceful

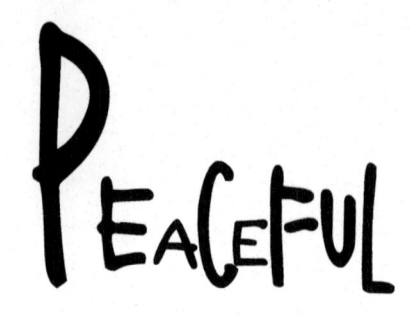

John 16:33
These things I have spoken to you, so that in Me you may have peace. In the world you have tribulation, but take courage; I have overcome the world. (NASB)

Isaiah 26:3
The Lord gives perfect peace to those whose faith is firm. (CEV)

John 14:27
I'm leaving you well and whole. That's My parting gift to you. Peace. I don't leave you the way you're used to being left—feeling abandoned, bereft. So don't be upset. Don't be distraught. (THE MESSAGE)

Colossians 3:15
The peace that Christ gives is to guide you in the decisions you make; for it is to this peace that God has called you together in the one body. And be thankful. (GNT)

Numbers 6:24-26
May the Lord bless you and take care of you; may the Lord be kind and gracious to you; may the Lord look on you with favor and give you peace. (GNT)

Situation:

_____
_____
_____
_____

Feelings:

_____
_____
_____
_____
_____

The lies that creep in about God:

_____
_____
_____
_____
_____

What GOD thinks of you:

_____
_____
_____
_____
_____
_____
_____

Pressure

Romans 12:2
And do not be conformed to this world, but be transformed by the renewing of your mind, so that you may prove what the will of God is, that which is good and acceptable and perfect. (NASB)

2 Corinthians 3:17
Now the Lord is the Spirit, and where the Spirit of the Lord is, there is liberty. (NIV)

2 Corinthians 6:14-18
Do not be yoked together with unbelievers. For what do righteousness and wickedness have in common? Or what fellowship can light have with darkness? What harmony is there between Christ and Belial? What does a believer have in common with an unbeliever? What agreement is there between the temple of God and idols? For we are the temple of the living God. As God has said: "I will live with them and walk among them, and I will be their God, and they will be My people. Therefore come out from them and be separate," says the Lord. "Touch no unclean thing, and I will receive you. I will be a Father to you, and you will be My sons and daughters," says the Lord Almighty. (NASB)

1 Thessalonians 5:5
You are all sons of the light and sons of the day. We do not belong to the night or to the darkness. So then, let us not be like others, who are asleep, but let us be alert and self-controlled. For those who sleep, sleep at night, and those who get drunk, get drunk at night. But since we belong to the day, let us be self-controlled, putting on faith and love as a breastplate, and the hope of salvation as a helmet. (NASB)

2 Corinthians 4:7-9
But we have this treasure in jars of clay to show that this all-surpassing power is from God and not from us. We are hard pressed on every side, but not crushed; perplexed, but not in despair; persecuted, but not abandoned; struck down, but not destroyed. (NASB)

Situation:

Feelings:

The lies that creep in about God:

What GOD thinks of you:

Quiet

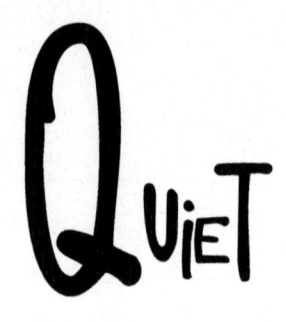

Psalm 23:2
He lets me rest in fields of green grass and leads me to quiet pools of fresh water. (GNT)

Isaiah 30:15
The holy Lord God of Israel had told all of you, "I will keep you safe if you turn back to Me and calm down. I will make you strong if you quietly trust Me." (CEV)

Exodus 14:13-14
But Moses said to the people, "Do not fear! Stand by and see the salvation of the LORD which He will accomplish for you today; for the Egyptians whom you have seen today, you will never see them again forever. The LORD will fight for you while you keep silent." (NASB)

Zephaniah 3:17
The LORD your God is in your midst, a victorious warrior. He will exult over you with joy, He will be quiet in His love, He will rejoice over you with shouts of joy. (NASB)

1 Peter 3:3-4
Your beauty should not come from outward adornment, such as elaborate hairstyles and the wearing of gold jewelry or fine clothes. Rather, it should be that of your inner self, the unfading beauty of a gentle and quiet spirit, which is of great worth in God's sight. (NIV)

Situation:

Feelings:

The lies that creep in about God:

What GOD thinks of you:

Rejected

1 Peter 2:4
Come to Jesus Christ. He is the living stone that people have rejected, but which God has chosen and highly honored. (CEV)

Matthew 21:42
Jesus replied, "You surely know that the Scriptures say, 'The stone that the builders tossed aside is now the most important stone of all. This is something the Lord has done, and it is amazing to us.'" (CEV)

1 Peter 2:9
But you are a chosen people, a royal priesthood, a holy nation, God's special possession, that you may declare the praises of Him who called you out of darkness into His wonderful light. (NIV)

Zechariah 10:6
I will make the people of Judah strong; I will rescue the people of Israel. I will have compassion on them and bring them all back home. They will be as though I had never rejected them. I am the Lord their God; I will answer their prayers. (GNT)

Romans 15:7
Honor God by accepting each other, as Christ has accepted you. (GNT)

Situation:

Feelings:

The lies that creep in about God:

What GOD thinks of you:

Revenge

Romans 12:19
Never take your own revenge, beloved, but leave room for God to defend you. For it is written, "Vengeance is Mine, I will repay," says the Lord. (NASB)

Luke 6:35
But love your enemies and be good to them. Lend without expecting to be paid back. Then you will get a great reward, and you will be the true children of God in heaven. He is good even to people who are unthankful and cruel. (CEV)

Zechariah 2:8
For this is what the Lord Almighty says: "After the Glorious One has sent me against the nations that have plundered you—for whoever touches you touches the apple of His eye." (NIV)

Psalm 35:19
Don't let my brutal enemies be glad because of me. They hate me for no reason. Don't let them wink behind my back. (CEV)

Proverbs 24:17-18
Do not gloat when your enemy falls; when they stumble, do not let your heart rejoice, or the Lord will see and disapprove and turn His wrath away from them. (NIV)

Situation:

Feelings:

The lies that creep in about God:

What GOD thinks of you:

Sadness

Isaiah 51:11
So the ransomed of the LORD will return and come with joyful shouting to Zion, and everlasting joy will be on their heads. They will obtain gladness and joy, and sorrow and sighing will flee away. (NASB)

Psalm 30:11-12
You turned my wailing into dancing; You removed my sackcloth and clothed me with joy, that my heart may sing to You and not be silent. O LORD my God, I will give You thanks forever. (NIV)

Psalm 27:6
Then my head will be exalted above the enemies who surround me; at His sacred tent I will sacrifice with shouts of joy; I will sing and make music to the Lord. (NIV)

Romans 14:17
For God's Kingdom is not a matter of eating and drinking, but of the righteousness, peace, and joy which the Holy Spirit gives. (GNT)

Romans 15:13
I pray that God, who gives hope, will bless you with complete happiness and peace because of your faith. And may the power of the Holy Spirit fill you with hope. (CEV)

Situation:

_____
_____
_____
_____
_____

Feelings:

_____
_____
_____
_____
_____
_____

The lies that creep in about God:

_____
_____
_____
_____
_____
_____

What GOD thinks of you:

_____
_____
_____
_____
_____
_____
_____
_____

Stupid

Romans 8:38-39
For I am convinced that neither death, nor life, nor angels, nor principalities, nor things present, nor things to come, nor powers, nor height, nor depth, nor any other created thing, will be able to separate us from the love of God, which is in Christ Jesus our Lord. (NASB)

Proverbs 3:5-7
Trust in the LORD with all your heart and do not lean on your own understanding. In all your ways acknowledge Him, and He will make your paths straight. Do not be wise in your own eyes; fear the LORD and turn away from evil. (NASB)

Proverbs 3:13-15
Blessed is the man who finds wisdom, the man who gains understanding, for she is more profitable than silver and yields better returns than gold. She is more precious than rubies; nothing you desire can compare with her. (NIV)

1 Corinthians 1:18-20
For the message about Christ's death on the cross is nonsense to those who are being lost; but for us who are being saved it is God's power. The Scripture says, "I will destroy the wisdom of the wise and set aside the understanding of the scholars." So then, where does that leave the wise? Or the scholars? Or the skillful debaters of this world? God has shown that this world's wisdom is foolishness! (GNT)

1 Corinthians 1:26-29
My dear friends, remember what you were when God chose you. The people of this world didn't think that many of you were wise. Only a few of you were in places of power, and not many of you came from important families. But God chose the foolish things of this world to put the wise to shame. He chose the weak things of this world to put the powerful to shame. What the world thinks is worthless, useless, and nothing at all is what God has used to destroy what the world considers important. God did all this to keep anyone from bragging to Him. (CEV)

Situation:

Feelings:

The lies that creep in about God:

What GOD thinks of you:

Thankful

Psalms 100:4
Enter His gates with thanksgiving and His courts with praise. (NASB)

Isaiah 51:3
Indeed, the LORD will comfort Zion; He will comfort all her waste places. And her wilderness He will make like Eden, and her desert like the garden of the LORD; joy and gladness will be found in her, thanksgiving and sound of a melody. (NASB)

Hebrews 13:5
Through Him then, let us continually offer up a sacrifice of praise to God, that is, the fruit of lips that give thanks to His name. (NASB)

Colossians 4:2
Pray diligently. Stay alert, with your eyes wide open in gratitude. (THE MESSAGE)

Revelation 7:11
All the angels were standing around the throne and around the elders and the four living creatures. They fell down on their faces before the throne and worshiped God, saying: "Amen! Praise and glory and wisdom and thanks and honor and power and strength be to our God for ever and ever. Amen!" (NIV)

Situation:

Feelings:

The lies that creep in about God:

What GOD thinks of you:

TROUBLED

John 11:33-36
When Jesus saw her weeping, and the Jews who had come along with her also weeping, He was deeply moved in spirit and troubled. "Where have you laid him?" He asked. "Come and see, Lord," they replied. Jesus wept. Then the Jews said, "See how He loved him!" (NIV)

1 Peter 1:6-9
In this you greatly rejoice, even though now for a little while, if necessary, you have been distressed by various trials, so that the proof of your faith, being more precious than gold which is perishable, even though tested by fire, may be found to result in praise and glory and honor at the revelation of Jesus Christ; and though you have not seen Him, you love Him, and though you do not see Him now, but believe in Him, you greatly rejoice with joy inexpressible and full of glory, obtaining as the outcome of your faith the salvation of your souls. (NASB)

John 12:27-28
"Now My heart is troubled—and what shall I say? Shall I say, 'Father, do not let this hour come upon Me'? But that is why I came—so that I might go through this hour of suffering. Father, bring glory to your name!" Then a voice spoke from heaven, "I have brought glory to it, and I will do so again." (GNT)

John 14:1-3
Don't let this throw you. You trust God, don't you? Trust Me. There is plenty of room for you in My Father's home. If that weren't so, would I have told you that I'm on My way to get a room ready for you? And if I'm on My way to get your room ready, I'll come back and get you so you can live where I live. (THE MESSAGE)

Psalm 9:9
The Lord is a refuge for the oppressed, a stronghold in times of trouble. Those who know Your name trust in You, for You, Lord, have never forsaken those who seek You. (NIV)

Situation:

Feelings:

The lies that creep in about God:

What GOD thinks of you:

Truthful

Colossians 3:9-10
Do not lie to one another, since you laid aside the old self with its evil practices, and have put on the new self who is being renewed to a true knowledge according to the image of the One who created him. (NASB)

Romans 3:4
Let God be true, and every human being a liar. (NIV)

2 Timothy 2:15
Be diligent to present yourself approved to God as a workman who does not need to be ashamed, accurately handling the word of truth. (NASB)

Hebrews 6:13-15
When God made His promise to Abraham, since there was no one greater for Him to swear by, He swore by Himself, saying, "I will surely bless you and give you many descendants." And so after waiting patiently, Abraham received what was promised. (NIV)

Psalm 40:10-11
I have not hidden Your righteousness within my heart; I have spoken of Your faithfulness and Your salvation; I have not concealed Your lovingkindness and Your truth from the great congregation. You, O Lord, will not withhold Your compassion from me; Your lovingkindness and Your truth will continually preserve me. (NASB)

Situation:

Feelings:

The lies that creep in about God:

What GOD thinks of you:

UGLY

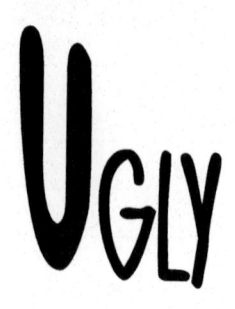

Psalm 139:13-18
You are the One who put me together inside my mother's body, and I praise You because of the wonderful way You created me. Everything You do is marvelous! Of this I have no doubt. Nothing about me is hidden from You! I was secretly woven together deep in the earth below, but with Your own eyes You saw my body being formed. Even before I was born, You had written in Your book everything I would do. Your thoughts are far beyond my understanding, much more than I could ever imagine. I try to count Your thoughts, but they outnumber the grains of sand on the beach. And when I awake, I will find You nearby. (CEV)

2 Corinthians 5:17
Anyone who belongs to Christ is a new person. The past is forgotten, and everything is new. (CEV)

Song of Solomon 7:6
How pretty you are, how beautiful; how complete the delights of your love. (GNT)

Psalm 17:8
Protect me as You would Your very own eyes; hide me in the shadow of Your wings. (CEV)

Zechariah 2:8
Anyone who strikes you strikes what is most precious to Me. (GNT)

Situation:

Feelings:

The lies that creep in about God:

What GOD thinks of you:

Understanding

Psalm 32:8-9
I will instruct you and teach you in the way you should go; I will counsel you and watch over you. Do not be like the horse or the mule, which have no understanding but must be controlled by bit and bridle or they will not come to you. (NIV)

1 Corinthians 2:14-16
The man without the Spirit does not accept the things that come from the Spirit of God, for they are foolishness to him, and he cannot understand them, because they are spiritually discerned. The spiritual man makes judgments about all things, but he himself is not subject to any man's judgment: "For who has known the mind of the Lord that he may instruct Him?" But we have the mind of Christ. (NIV)

1 John 5:20
We know that the Son of God has come and has given us understanding, so that we know the true God. We live in union with the true God—in union with His Son Jesus Christ. This is the true God, and this is eternal life. (GNT)

Ephesians 6:1-3
Children, you belong to the Lord, and you do the right thing when you obey your parents. The first commandment with a promise says, "Obey your father and your mother, and you will have a long and happy life." (CEV)

Proverbs 1:7-10
The fear of the LORD is the beginning of knowledge; fools despise wisdom and instruction. Hear, my son, your father's instruction and do not forsake your mother's teaching; indeed, they are a graceful wreath to your head and ornaments about your neck. My son, if sinners entice you, do not consent. (NASB)

Situation:

Feelings:

The lies that creep in about God:

What GOD thinks of you:

Unworthy

Luke 18:13-14
But the tax collector stood at a distance. He would not even look up to heaven, but beat his breast and said, "God, have mercy on me, a sinner." I tell you that this man, rather than the other, went home justified before God. For everyone who exalts himself will be humbled, and he who humbles himself will be exalted. (NIV)

Ephesians 2:8-10
For by grace you have been saved through faith; and that not of yourselves, it is the gift of God; not as a result of works, so that no one may boast. For we are His workmanship, created in Christ Jesus for good works, which God prepared beforehand so that we would walk in them. (NASB)

2 Peter 1:8-9
For if these qualities are yours and are increasing, they render you neither useless nor unfruitful in the true knowledge of our Lord Jesus Christ. For he who lacks these qualities is blind or short-sighted, having forgotten his purification from his former sins. (NASB)

Romans 4:4-5
Money paid to workers isn't a gift. It is something they earn by working. But you cannot make God accept you because of something you do. God accepts sinners only because they have faith in Him. (CEV)

Colossians 1:9-10
For this reason we have always prayed for you, ever since we heard about you. We ask God to fill you with the knowledge of His will, with all the wisdom and understanding that His Spirit gives. Then you will be able to live as the Lord wants and will always do what pleases Him. Your lives will produce all kinds of good deeds, and you will grow in your knowledge of God. (GNT)

Situation:

Feelings:

The lies that creep in about God:

What GOD thinks of you:

Victorious

Zechariah 3:17
The Lord your God is with you; His power gives you victory. The Lord will take delight in you, and in His love He will give you new life. He will sing and be joyful over you. (GNT)

Exodus 15:1-2
Moses and the Israelites sang this song in praise of the Lord: "I sing praises to the Lord for His great victory! He has thrown the horses and their riders into the sea. The Lord is my strength, the reason for my song, because He has saved me. I praise and honor the Lord—He is my God and the God of my ancestors. (CEV)

Philippians 4:12-13
I know what it is to be in need, and I know what it is to have plenty. I have learned the secret of being content in any and every situation, whether well fed or hungry, whether living in plenty or in want. I can do everything through Him who gives me strength. (NIV)

Proverbs 11:14
For lack of guidance a nation falls, but victory is won through many advisers. (NIV)

Proverbs 21:31
The horse is prepared for the day of battle, but victory belongs to the LORD. (NASB)

1 Corinthians 15:57
But thanks be to God who gives us the victory through our Lord Jesus Christ! (GNT)

Situation:

Feelings:

The lies that creep in about God:

What GOD thinks of you:

WAITING

Proverbs 8:33-35
Listen to what you are taught. Be wise; do not neglect it. Those who listen to me will be happy—those who stay at my door every day, waiting at the entrance to my home. Those who find me find life, and the Lord will be pleased with them. (GNT)

2 Chronicles 16:9
For the eyes of the Lord range throughout the earth to strengthen those whose hearts are fully committed to Him. (NIV)

Jude 1:21
Dear friends, keep building on the foundation of your most holy faith, as the Holy Spirit helps you to pray. And keep in step with God's love, as you wait for our Lord Jesus Christ to show how kind He is by giving you eternal life. (CEV)

Psalm 27:14
Wait for the LORD; be strong and let your heart take courage. Yes, wait for the LORD. (NASB)

Psalm 37:7
Rest in the LORD and wait patiently for Him; do not fret because of him who prospers in his way, because of the man who carries out wicked schemes. (NASB)

Situation:

Feelings:

The lies that creep in about God:

What GOD thinks of you:

Wisdom

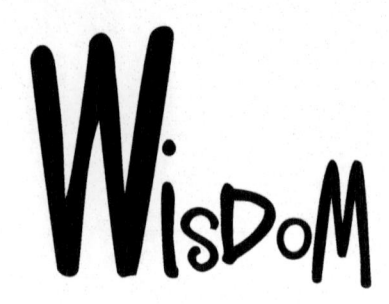

Proverbs 1:20
Wisdom shouts in the street, she lifts her voice in the square; at the head of the noisy streets she cries out; at the entrance of the gates in the city she utters her sayings: "How long, O naive ones, will you love being simple-minded? And scoffers delight themselves in scoffing and fools hate knowledge? Turn to my reproof, behold, I will pour out my spirit on you; I will make my words known to you." (NASB)

Proverbs 2:10-13
You will become wise, and your knowledge will give you pleasure. Your insight and understanding will protect you and prevent you from doing the wrong thing. They will keep you away from people who stir up trouble by what they say—those who have abandoned a righteous life to live in the darkness of sin. (GNT)

James 1:5
But if any of you lacks wisdom, let him ask God, who gives to all generously and without reproach, and it will be given to you. (NASB)

James 3:17
But the wisdom that comes from above leads us to be pure, friendly, gentle, sensible, kind, helpful, genuine, and sincere. (CEV)

Colossians 1:9-12
For this reason, since the day we heard about you, we have not stopped praying for you and asking God to fill you with the knowledge of His will through all spiritual wisdom and understanding. And we pray this in order that you may live a life worthy of the Lord and may please Him in every way: bearing fruit in every good work, growing in the knowledge of God, being strengthened with all power according to His glorious might so that you may have great endurance and patience, and joyfully giving thanks to the Father, who has qualified you to share in the inheritance of the saints in the kingdom of light. (NIV)

Situation:

Feelings:

The lies that creep in about God:

What GOD thinks of you:

Worry

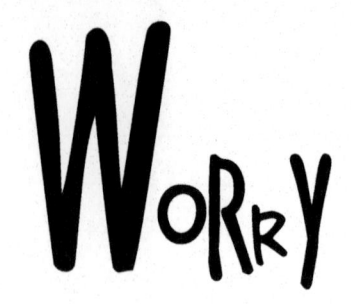

Psalm 46:10-11
Cease striving and know that I am God; I will be exalted among the nations, I will be exalted in the earth. The LORD of hosts is with us; the God of Jacob is our stronghold. (NASB)

Matthew 6:34
Don't worry about tomorrow. It will take care of itself. You have enough to worry about today. (CEV)

Jeremiah 29:11
I alone know the plans I have for you, plans to bring you prosperity and not disaster, plans to bring about the future you hope for. (GNT)

Philippians 4:6
Be anxious for nothing, but in everything by prayer and supplication with thanksgiving let your requests be made known to God. And the peace of God, which surpasses all comprehension, will guard your hearts and your minds in Christ Jesus. (NASB)

Philippians 4:19
And my God will meet all your needs according to the riches of His glory in Christ Jesus. (NIV)

1 Peter 5:7
God cares for you, so turn all your worries over to Him. (CEV)

Situation:

Feelings:

The lies that creep in about God:

What GOD thinks of you:

EXCITED

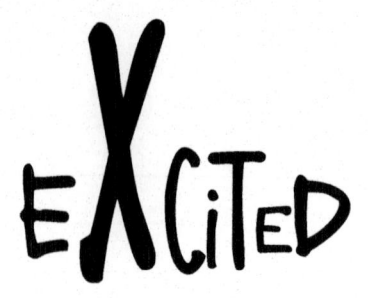

1 Peter 1:8
And though you have not seen Him, you love Him, and though you do not see Him now, but believe in Him, you greatly rejoice with joy inexpressible and full of glory. (NASB)

2 Corinthians 9:15
Thank God for this gift, His gift. No language can praise it enough! (THE MESSAGE)

Romans 15:13
Now may the God of hope fill you with all joy and peace in believing, so that you will abound in hope by the power of the Holy Spirit. (NASB)

Romans 5:3-5
Not only so, but we also glory in our sufferings, because we know that suffering produces perseverance; perseverance, character; and character, hope. And hope does not put us to shame, because God's love has been poured out into our hearts through the Holy Spirit, who has been given to us. (NIV)

Psalm 5:11
Let all who run to You for protection always sing joyful songs. Provide shelter for those who truly love You and let them rejoice. (CEV)

Situation:

Feelings:

The lies that creep in about God:

What GOD thinks of you:

Yielded

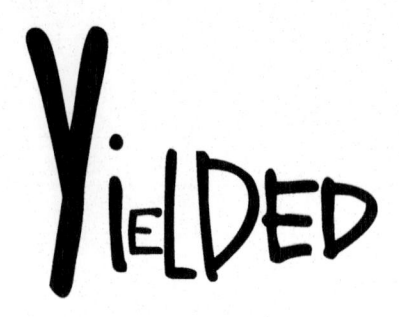

James 4:7
So then, submit yourselves to God. Resist the devil, and he will run away from you. (GNT)

Psalm 112:1
Praise the LORD! How blessed is the man who fears the LORD, who greatly delights in His commandments. (NASB)

Proverbs 4:13
Take firm hold of instruction, do not let go; guard her, for she is your life. (AMP)

Proverbs 3:5-6
Trust in the Lord with all your heart and lean not on your own understanding; in all your ways submit to Him, and He will make your paths straight. (NIV)

Philippians 2:12-13
Therefore, my dear friends, as you have always obeyed—not only in my presence, but now much more in my absence—continue to work out your salvation with fear and trembling, for it is God who works in you to will and to act in order to fulfill His good purpose. (NIV)

Situation:

_____
_____
_____
_____
_____

Feelings:

_____
_____
_____
_____
_____

The lies that creep in about God:

_____
_____
_____
_____
_____

What GOD thinks of you:

_____
_____
_____
_____
_____
_____
_____

Zeal

Philippians 3:7-8
But Christ has shown me that what I once thought was valuable is worthless. Nothing is as wonderful as knowing Christ Jesus my Lord. I have given up everything else and count it all as garbage. All I want is Christ. (CEV)

Hebrews 12:1
Therefore, since we have so great a cloud of witnesses surrounding us, let us also lay aside every encumbrance and the sin which so easily entangles us, and let us run with endurance the race that is set before us. (NASB)

1 Corinthians 2:2
For I resolved to know nothing while I was with you except Jesus Christ and Him crucified. (NIV)

John 2:14-17
In the temple courts He found people selling cattle, sheep and doves, and others sitting at tables exchanging money. So He made a whip out of cords, and drove all from the temple courts, both sheep and cattle; He scattered the coins of the moneychangers and overturned their tables. To those who sold doves He said, "Get these out of here! Stop turning My Father's house into a market!" His disciples remembered that it is written: "Zeal for Your house will consume Me." (NIV)

I Corinthians 2:9-10
But just as it is written, "Things which eye has not seen and ear has not heard, and which have not entered the heart of man, all that God has prepared for those who love Him." For to us God revealed them through the Spirit; for the Spirit searches all things, even the depths of God. (NASB)

Situation:

Feelings:

The lies that creep in about God:

What GOD thinks of you:

Terri Fornear is a Licensed Language Therapist and Family and Individual Life Coach. For 25 years, she has worked with children, teenagers and adults to help them face emotions that have blocked academic, relational, social and spiritual success.

In 2008, Terri co-founded Stronghold Ministry with her husband, Joe. Stronghold is a nonprofit organization which helps cancer patients and those in crisis to discover God's salvation, truth and love in the midst of difficult times. Out of the depths of her own experiences and challenges—lifelong learning differences, her husband's near-death battle with Stage IV cancer in 2003 and being a pastor's wife for 18 years—she has navigated a range of life's emotions.

In this journal, Terri helps identify the lies about God that hinder us from being all that He lovingly created us to be. The key is to quickly replace thoughts which paralyze us with truths about God—truths that are lifted straight from the pages of God's Word to us. This journal is a tool that penetrates dark emotions to transfer us into the freedom and joy of God's truth and light.

Contact Information for Terri Fornear

E-mail
tfor@mystronghold.org

Phone
469-628-8192

Terri (and Joe) Fornear's blog
www.mystronghold.org/Blog/

Website
www.mystronghold.org

Mailing address
Stronghold Ministry
P.O. Box 38478
Dallas, TX 75238
214-221-2007

Information on Stronghold Ministry

Stronghold Ministry was founded by Joe and Terri Fornear to provide spiritual support and comfort to cancer patients, caretakers and others in major life crisis. We reach out through personal contact, through the Internet and via telephone. Please don't hesitate to call us or to refer someone who wants or needs some spiritual help! We want to be in your corner!

Services

We provide counseling; host support groups; and speak in home groups, Sunday school classes and youth groups. Joe is available as a guest speaker at your church service, and we host retreats and conferences as well.

We offer our services free to cancer patients and those in crisis. Stronghold Ministry operates solely on donations. We have incorporated as a nonprofit in the State of Texas and have been granted 501(c) 3 tax exemption status by the IRS, so donations are tax deductible. Stronghold Ministry has chosen to join ECFA, The Evangelical Council for Financial Accountability, which oversees the financial practices of nonprofit organizations.

NOTES

NOTES

CPSIA information can be obtained
at www.ICGtesting.com
Printed in the USA
FSOW04n0503010615
7466FS

9 780984 011322